Hidden medical benefits of sex for couples

Reduces stress

Burns calories

Boosts immunity

Lowers blood pressure

Reduces risk of prostate cancer

Sex anxiety

Fear of sex and it causes

Consequences of sex rejection

Remedies for sex phobia

Laurence Payne

Copyright©2022 Sonia Radley

All right Reserved

INTRODUCTION

CHAPTER ONE

MEDICAL BENEFITS OF SEX:
THESE ARE SOME OF THE SECRET ADVANTAGES OF HAVING INTERCOURSE
1. Decreases pressure
2. Gives your skin a sparkle
3. Further develops rest
4. Get Less Colds and Boost Your Immune System
5. Ease period torment
6. Help Your Libido
7. Work on Women's Bladder Control
8. Work on Women's Bladder Control
10. Considers Exercise
11. Lower Heart Attack Risk
12. Decrease Pain

CHAPTER TWO

THE EXACT NUMBER OF CALORIES THAT CAN BE CONSUMED DURING VARIOUS SEX POSITIONS
2. An exotic back rub
3. Missionary position
4. Ladies on top - cowgirl position
5. doggy style
6. Invert cowgirl
7. The plow
8. The ascent passion

CHAPTER THREE

REASONS BEHIND WHY YOU OUGHT TO HAVE INTERCOURSE WITH YOUR PARTNER EACH DAY

CHAPTER FOUR

5 Health Benefits of Kissing your companion

CHAPTER FIVE

The medical benefits of having sex with your pregnant lady
1 It brings down circulatory strain
2 Labor and recovery are less troublesome
3 Stress alleviation
4 Stronger ties
5 Fewer visits to the bathroom
6 preventing complication

CHAPTER SIX

There are various kinds of dismissal
Reasons inspired by a paranoid fear of sex

CHAPTER SEVEN

Ordinary phobic responses include
Treatment for Genophobia
When to see a specialist

CHAPTER EIGHT

Diagnosing fear of intimacy
Beating trepidation of intimacy

Grappling with your apprehension about intimacy
Esteem yourself
Impart
Look for help from an expert
At the point when your partner fears intimacy
Focus point

CHAPTER NINE

The connection between uneasiness and sex
How to lighten sex tension?
Converse with your primary care physician
Investigate intimacy in various ways
Be careful
Make sex a customary discussion
Try not to limit foreplay
Investigate issues of disgrace
Look for proficient assistance
Facing everyday life after sexual uneasiness
Conclusion

Introduction

This book titled "hidden medical benefits" of sex for couples is a manual composed and suggested for spouses who are looking for a glow in their relationship. This book targets assisting couples with resuscitating closeness and light the flash in their relationship. Sex is one of the mainstays of marriage and any reasonable person would agree that it is a significant point of support in fruitful relationships. This assertion is questionable as individuals have alternate points of view about existence and what is vital to one isn't altogether considered to be vital to the next.

Sex isn't always necessary, yet it tends to be a significant piece of a sound satisfying relationship. How significant it is can change starting with one individual then onto the next.

Certain individuals might feel that having a sexual association with their partner is crucial. Others might feel that different sorts of closeness and association are more significant.

A portion of the reasons that you may feel that sex is important in a relationship incorporates;

- Feeling nearer to your partner
- Showing fondness to your partner
- when you consider it to be fun and pleasurable
- A craving to have children
- Feeling sure and provocative

- Soothing pressure

The research proposes that having successive sex can assume a part in more love. At the point when couples experience more warmth, they are additionally bound to then have more incessant sex upholds a sound relationship in various ways, for example, the oxytocin delivered during sex upgrades a feeling of holding and works on enthusiastic closeness.

Sex is a monogamous relationship that builds your degree of responsibility and enthusiastic association with the other individual. Communicating love through sex improves the probability of couples remaining together. Subsequently, sex is decidedly connected with a lower divorce rate.

Things being what they are, on the off chance that you are frequently down with a cold? Disregard hot chicken soup and have a few hot activities between the sheets. Indeed, the climax isn't the main advantage of sex, it is likewise really great for your wellbeing. Aside from reinforcing your security with your partner, having intercourse will work on your invulnerability, decrease tension and work on your general wellbeing. Peruse on to know more secret advantages of sex.

This book reveals insight into the various advantages of sex and the way that it is essential to wellbeing which can likewise help the life span of relationships. To be with one another for quite a while, the two of them would need to be in a decent spot intellectually and wellbeing shrewd.

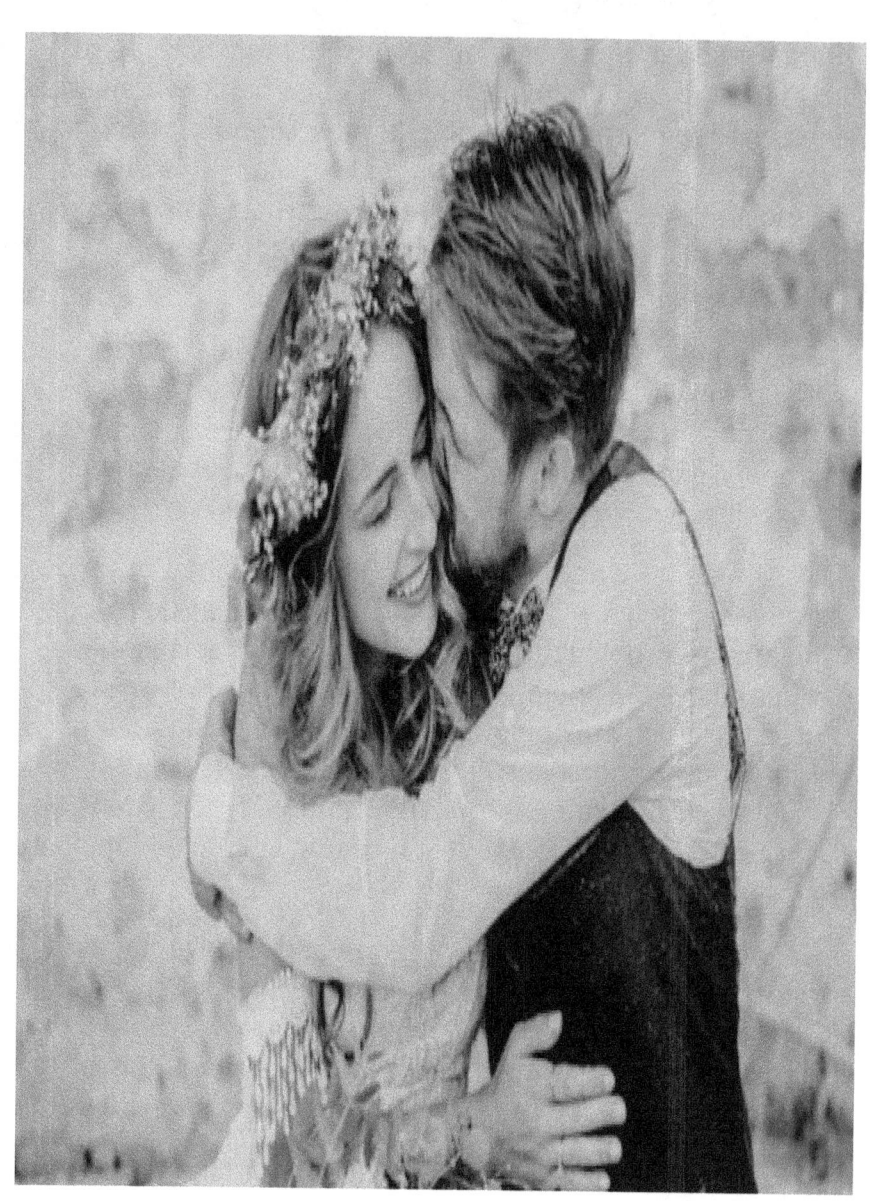

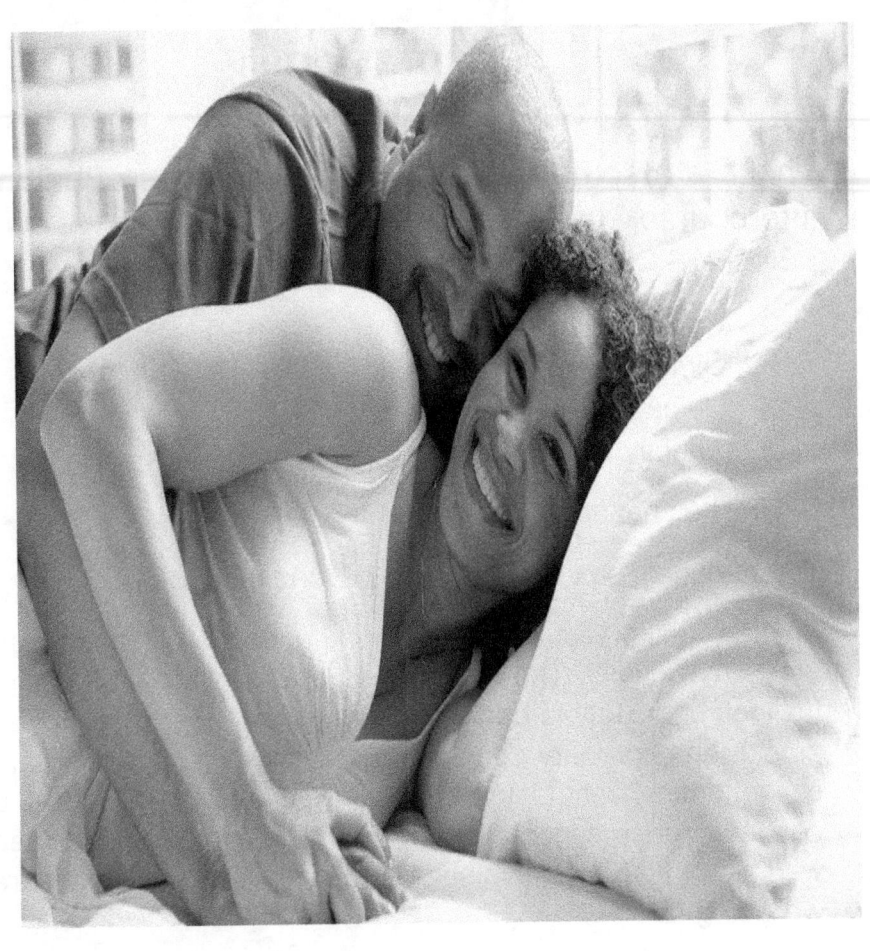

Chapter one
Medical benefits of sex:

These are some of the secret advantages of having intercourse

BENEFITS OF SEX (what can keep you solid is sex]

- Consumes calories
- Diminishes pressure
- Helps insusceptibility
- Brings down pulse

Diminishes hazard of prostate disease

The benefit of sex expands well beyond the room...

Sex isn't just pleasurable; did you know it's additionally great for you? It's valid. The advantages of sex range from cutting feelings of anxiety to bringing down your danger of malignant growth and coronary episodes. Sex works with touching and sensations of intimacy with your companion. This sort of connectedness accomplishes more than causes you to feel warm and fluffy, it diminishes tension and lifts your general wellbeing.

1. Decreases pressure

Sex is an incredible pressure reliever. That is because contacting, embracing, sexual closeness, and enthusiastic connection invigorate the arrival of "feel better" substances that advance holding and serenity. Sexual excitement additionally delivers substances that invigorate the prize and joy framework in the mind. Cultivating closeness and closeness can assist with diminishing nervousness and lift in general wellbeing.

Kissing and touching delivery feel-great chemicals, which will quiet you down. Also having intercourse discharges synthetics that will touch off your cerebrum's pleasure mind and will ease the pressure. Your body will be overwhelmed by the alleviating chemical when you have a climax. It will help your confidence and certainty. Thus, next time you have a meeting, consider slipping between the sheets before taking off.

2. Gives your skin a sparkle

As indicated by a review, the individuals who were making out somewhere around four times each week were looking seven to 12 years more youthful than their real age. In this way, get going with your accomplice to look youthful. Sex discharges chemicals like estrogen and testosterone, which assist you with looking youthful. It additionally smoothens out the kinks. The arrival of estrogen makes your hair sparkly and skin delicate. Ladies past their menopausal age have more kinks and dry skin as their estrogen level plunges. Having intercourse will deliver the chemical, which is valuable for them.

3. Further develops rest

Sex can assist you with dozing better. That is on the basis that climax procreates the appearance of a chemical called prolactin, a characteristic tranquilizer. Prolactin advances sensations of unwinding and sluggishness. This is only one reason you might see that you make some more straightforward memories nodding off after engaging in sexual relations.

Try not to fault your accomplice assuming he rests off just in the wake of making out. It happens because after climax a chemical called prolactin is delivered to your body. This chemical is answerable for languor. It will likewise make you looser.

4. Get Less Colds and Boost Your Immune System

More sex approaches fewer days off. That is what the aftereffects of studies contrasting physically dynamic individuals with the people who are not physically dynamic say. Sex supports your body's capacity to make defensive antibodies against microbes, infections, and different microorganisms that cause normal diseases. There's something else to developing a powerful invulnerable framework besides having a solid sexual coexistence. Eating right, working out, getting satisfactory rest, and staying up with the latest inoculations all add to having solid and sound guards against infectious sicknesses.

Getting hot and sweat-soaked between the sheets will assist you with forestalling a typical virus. Engaging in sexual relations has been found to build the degree of immunoglobulin A, a counter-acting agent. This immunizer will assist you with combatting the normal cold and influenza.

5. Ease period torment

Tune in up, women! Engage in sexual relations to facilitate your feminine spasms. During a spasm, uterus muscle contracts, and having a hot meeting with your accomplice has displayed to calm the pressure in the muscles. Sex during your period might appear to be muddled and a piece unappealing, yet you can deal with that by resting on a dim shaded towel.

6. Help Your Libido

In all honesty, the best cure for melting-away moxie is to engage in sexual relations! Engaging in sexual relations helps want. What's more on the off chance that aggravation and vaginal dryness make it trying for certain ladies to have intercourse, sexual action can assist with combatting these issues, as well. Sex helps vaginal oil, bloodstream to the vagina, and flexibility of the tissues, all of which make for better, more pleasurable sex and uplifted moxie.

7. Work on Women's Bladder Control
Urinary incontinence influences around 30% of ladies' sooner or later throughout everyday life. Having normal orgasm makes a woman's pelvic floor muscles work, reinforcing and conditioning them. Climaxes enact the very muscles that ladies use while doing Kegel works out. When your pelvic muscle is sensible it indicates that there's less danger of mishaps and pee spills.

8. Work on Women's Bladder Control
Urinary incontinence influences around 30% of ladies eventually throughout everyday life. Having customary climaxes works a lady's pelvic floor muscles, reinforcing and conditioning them. Climaxes initiate the very muscles that ladies use while doing Kegel works out.

Sex brings down your circulatory strain.

9. Bring down Your Blood Pressure Might it be said that you are one of the large numbers of individuals who experience the ill effects of hypertension? Sex can help you with taking it down. Many examinations have recorded a connection between intercourse explicitly (not masturbation) and lower systolic pulse, the principal number that shows up on a circulatory strain test. That is uplifting news for people searching for a simple aide to the way of life (diet, work out, stress decrease) and medicine methodologies to get the pulse into a solid reach. Sex meetings can't supplant

circulatory strain bringing drugs down to control hypertension, however, they might be a helpful expansion.

10. Considers Exercise

Like every other sort of active work, sex consumes calories, as well! Squatting and gazing at the TV use up around 1 calorie each moment. When you engage in sexual relations it builds your pulse and uses different muscle gatherings, consuming around 5 calories each moment. Normal sex can't supplant meetings at the rec center, however, having a functioning, sound sexual coexistence is a great method for getting some extra active work.

11. Lower Heart Attack Risk

Need a better heart? Have more sex. Sexual movements can helps keep some levels of hormones, similar to estrogen and testosterone, within proper limits. In check. when the hormones are out of balance, conditions like coronary illness and osteoporosis might create. When it comes to securing heart health by having sex, more is better. One review in men showed that the individuals who had intercourse somewhere around 2 times each week were half less inclined to pass on from coronary illness than their less physically dynamic friends.

12. Decrease Pain

Sexual feeling (counting masturbation) and climax can assist with keeping torment under control. The two exercises can decrease torment sensation and increment your aggravation edge. Climaxes bring about the arrival of chemicals that can assist with hindering torment signals. Some women report that self-stimulation through masturbation can decrease manifestations of menstrual cramps, joint inflammation, and even cerebral pain.

13. May Reduce Prostate Cancer Risk

There are male-explicit medical benefits of sex, as well. One review showed that men who had incessant discharges (characterized as 21 times each month or more) were less inclined to foster prostate disease than the people who had fewer discharges. It didn't make any difference on the off chance that the discharges happened through intercourse, masturbation, or nighttime outflows.

There's something else to prostate malignant growth hazard besides the recurrence of discharges, however, this was one intriguing finding.

14. Consume Calories

Sex can be used as a rundown of exercises that consumes calories. One review in children and ladies showed that sex consumes around 108 calories each half hour! That is to the point of consuming off 3, 570 calories - that is somewhat more than the number of calories in a single pound - in 32 half-hour meetings.

15. Reinforce Your Well-Being

People are wired for the social association. Connection with loved ones helps your general wellbeing and prosperity. Close associations with others, including your accomplice, make you more joyful and better contrasted with the individuals who are less all-around associated. Studies demonstrate it!

16. Further develop Intimacy and Relationships

You can embrace and nestle your method for growing warm, close connections. Sex and climaxes invigorate the arrival of a chemical called oxytocin that assists individuals' withholding. This "adoration chemical" as it's generally known, helps fabricate sensations of affection and trust. In an investigation of premenopausal ladies, the additional time the women spent canoodling and embracing their spouses or accomplices, the higher their oxytocin levels were. The chemical motivates fluffy sentiments and liberality, as well.

17. Look Younger

Forget surgery and anti-aging cream, sex keeps you more youthful-looking, as well. regular sex stimulates the arrival of estrogen and testosterone, chemicals that keep you younger and indispensable looking. Estrogen advances more youthful-looking skin and shiny locks. In one study, judges viewed participants in a one-way mirror and guessed their ages. Individuals who had intercourse something like 4 times each week with a standard accomplice were seen to be 7 to 12 years more youthful than they were.

18. Live Longer

What's the key to living longer? It could be having more sex. In a very long-term investigation of more than 1,000 moderately aged men, the individuals who had the most climaxes had a large portion of the demise pace of the people who didn't discharge habitually. Many elements add to life span, however having a functioning sexual coexistence might be a simple, pleasurable method for expanding your life expectancy.

19. Support Brainpower

Sex extends a lot of medical benefits from head to toe. A functioning sexual coexistence may make your cerebrum work better. Analysts observed that sex switches the mind into a more scientific method of and remembering to process. Also, animal studies recommend that sex enhances the region of the brain engaged in memory.

20. Sex Makes Fertilization Easier

With regards to growing your family, careful discipline brings about promising results. A review performed at a fruitfulness community observed that men who had day-by-day discharges for seven days had better sperm than the people who didn't discharge day by day. Men in the everyday discharge bunch had sperm with DNA that was less divided than the DNA from sperm of men who discharged less oftentimes. Less divided DNA suggests better DNA. Furthermore, good sperm that have solid DNA are bound to prepare an egg.

Chapter two
The exact number of calories that can be consumed during various sex positions

We as a whole expertise significant exercise is to remain fit and sound, yet here and there the exercise routine becomes exhausting. In this way, when you are not in the mindset to work it out in the rec center, then, at that point, have a sweat-soaked meeting in your home with your partner. No, we are not looking at practicing together, yet a more pleasant action that will likewise assist you with burning those additional Calories-Sex. Furthermore, with sex, we mean everything from kisses, foreplay, and all the other things. It isn't only extraordinary for your relationship yet in addition for your wellbeing. You will want to consume off the calories from your after-supper sweet treat with simply thirty minutes of enthusiastic lovemaking meetings with your partner. A few muscle bunches are involved when you engage in sexual relations. To know the number of calories you consume when you and your partner are attempting different sex positions and heartfelt exercises.

1. *Smooching*

For certain calories to consume, you want to kiss as you did during the underlying phases of your relationship, where the lip-lock continued for the greater part of 60 minutes. That is the sort of kiss that will keep your relationship solid, work on your bond with your accomplice and assist you with consuming some fat. You can consume very nearly 90 calories if your kisses are lively and amaze you. To consolidate your kissing meeting with practices then, at that point, take a stab at kissing in a strange position like kissing him while doing pushups. You will consume 171 calories by doing pushups quickly.

2. An exotic back rub

Get some downtime for love-making and think about giving an arousing back rub to your accomplice. It won't just hotness things up, however, you will likewise consume a few calories. A decent rubdown is generally welcome and if you are giving the back rub, move slowly, to make it a more erotic and compelling exercise. You will be drawing in various muscles while going more slowly.

3. Missionary position

Minister position is the point at which two or three have intercourse confronting one another and the lady is under the man. You will consume around 50 to 60 calories during a 30-minute meeting. Women, you can make this hotter and compelling by doing some hip development. You can likewise add murmuring and little groaning for some, additional calorie consumption.

4. Ladies on top - cowgirl position

A few women love this situation as it offers more satisfaction and a noteworthy peak. It is likewise an extraordinary exercise for your gluteus muscles and thighs. Squat on top of your accomplice and add a little hip development with skipping all over to get your heart hustling. This position will assist you with burning around 200 calories quickly.

5. doggy style

As indicated by a review led by the National Survey of Family Growth, only 36% of ladies and 44 percent of men have attempted the pup sex position to some degree once. It is probably the best situation to hit the G-spot. This sex position is preferred by practically every one of the men and by ladies who like it profoundly. From the rear intercourse will consume around 100 to 105 calories in a short time.

6. Invert cowgirl

This is a variety of the lady on top position or cowgirl position. Here, the young lady faces the person. Have your accomplice rests and afterward squat over him confronting his feet. Young ladies like this situation as it makes them responsible for the entrance and speed. This position causes her to feel sexier. A converse cowgirl position will assist you with consuming around 280 calories in an 80-minute meeting.

7. The plow

The furrow position includes the lady lying on her stomach with the person remaining between her legs and raising the lady's thighs for profound infiltration. Even though it is an interesting position, it is an incredible exercise for your center and arms. You will consume almost 64 calories in a moment.

8. The ascent passion

This standing position is an in-your-face exercise for the man. In the rising to energy position, the man and the lady remain to confront one another. The man then, at that point, lifts the lady for entrance and the lady simply folds her legs over him or keeps them on the bed or couch behind him. This position will assist you with consuming around 67 calories in a moment and it draws in your leg muscles, calves, gluteus, and arms.

You can consume an additional 60 to 100 calories by arriving at the climax. Furthermore, to make your sex meeting an exercise meeting, make it all the wilder and more energetic.

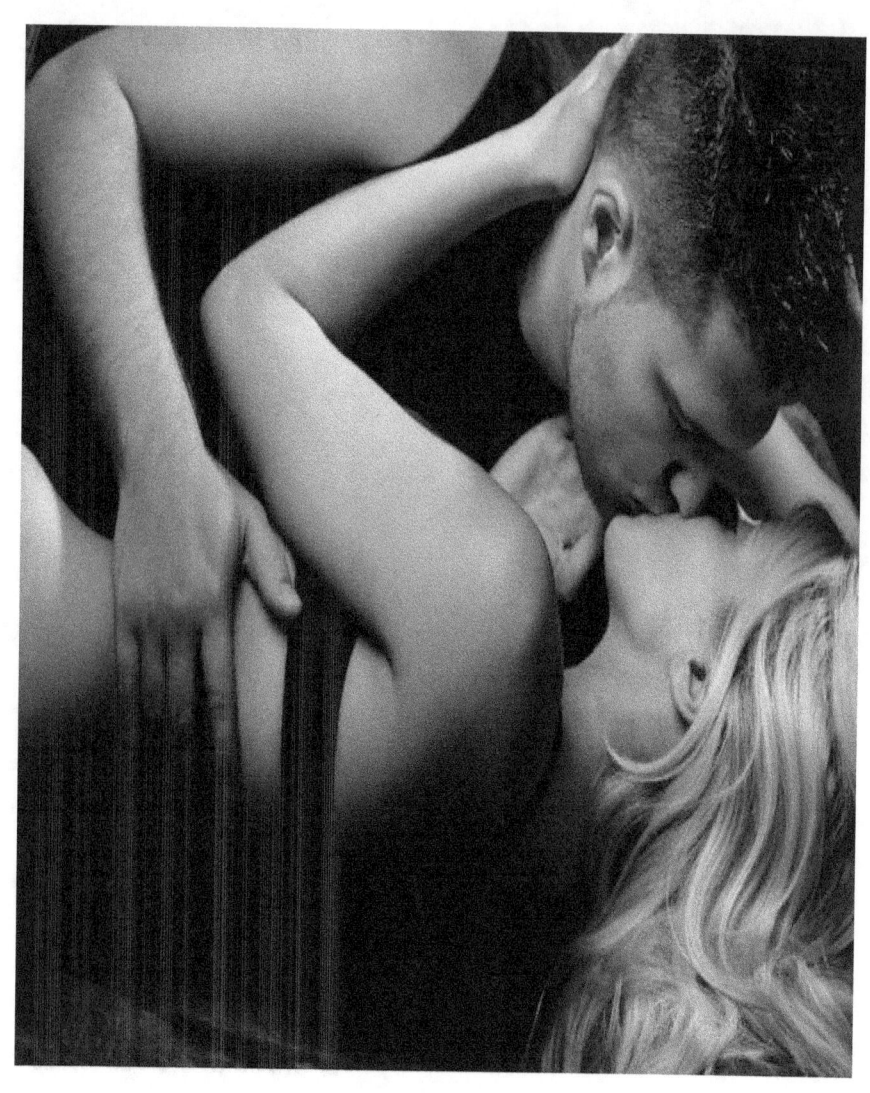

Chapter three

reasons behind why you ought to have intercourse with your partner each day

Getting intimate with your partner can be possible whenever you want to at any time of the day. It's vital to realize that there are a ton of medical advantages, of getting personal with your accomplice toward the beginning of the day. This article will see four reasons, why you ought to get close with your accomplice each day.

This includes the following

1 it helps you not to be worried and it advances holding with your accomplice. Having intercourse with your accomplice gives out chemicals called endorphins, which cause you to feel blissful. It likewise gives out another chemical called oxytocin, which assuages pressure and makes you lose. It can likewise assist you in withholding with your accomplice.

2 it assists you with consuming calories

Having intercourse with your accomplice toward the beginning of the day can likewise fill in as an exercise. As per research, having intercourse consumes five calories each moment, when you participate in it for certain minutes, you can consume a ton of calories.

3 it supports your safe framework

Getting private with your accomplice toward the beginning of the day can build your resistant framework. It exercises your body's guard framework against microorganisms and infections.

4 it is great for your cerebrum

Getting private with your accomplice toward the beginning of the day assists with supporting your intellectual ability. At the point when you participate in closeness with your accomplice, your body gives out chemicals like dopamine which is helpful for your mental wellbeing and cognizance.

Chapter four

5 Health Benefits of Kissing your companion

Kissing is a characteristic impulse for people and the most unconstrained presentation of warmth. A long kiss on the lips is comparably critical in a man-lady relationship to foster security, holding, and friendship, much as a child has a solid sense of reassurance in a mother's warm embrace followed by a long kiss on the cheek. Kissing is a typical approach to communicating adoration and want.

Kissing has a lot of medical benefits also. Kissing is supposed to be a disposition enhancer, a releaser of significant chemicals, and perhaps the best lifestyle choice for a solid and blissful life. Kissing is helpful to your well-being.

1 To dispose of those additional calories, give a kiss

There is no compelling reason to go to the exercise center to get thinner and get in shape. Going through just a few minutes kissing your adored one will bring about a 6 calorie misfortune.

Consider the number of calories you will save from a powerful kissing meeting with your darling. Kissing speeds up your body digestion permitting you to consume calories with less exertion. Would you be able to accept that kissing could have such a medical advantage?

2 Bid goodbye to a throbbing painfulness

At the point when you kiss, the pressure in your nerves and veins is delivered, which expands blood dissemination all through the body. Agonies, migraines, and different kinds of spasms in your body can be effortlessly treated after the strain is diminished and your veins grow.

As recently said, serotonin causes you to feel tranquil, and it can significantly help you assume that you are anxious for whatever purpose. Kissing has a quieting impact on your mindset vacillations also. So if your adored one is in torment, kiss the person in question as well as the other way around.

3 kissing can give you a more youthful appearance

Kissing incorporates the use of around 112 postural muscles and 34 face muscles, as per science when you kiss, your muscles become conditioned and prepared so that you show up much preferable and more youthful over common.

4 kissing can keep your teeth stay solid

On account of the vibe of kissing, the causticity connected with tooth depressions is killed by expanded spit creation in the mouth. Furthermore, the additional salivation washes away plaque that has developed in the mouth, spit's mineral salt part regularly assists with ensuring tooth polish.

5 kissing has been displayed to further develop heart wellbeing since it alleviates pressure, which is often contemplations to be the central reason for coronary illness.

Kissing likewise brings down cholesterol levels and brings pulse due down to the widening of veins that happen during the demonstration of kissing. Generally, kissing is related to a sound heart.

Chapter five

The medical benefits of having sex with your pregnant lady

At the point when you're pregnant, sex may be the thing at the forefront of your thoughts, with the creation of a portion of your going chemicals, morning ailment, and always growing waistline. Having intercourse can do ponders for your wellbeing, pregnancy, and relationship.

The following are six motivations behind why engaging in sexual relations during pregnancy is sound both genuinely and intellectually.

1 It brings down circulatory strain

Although your pulse might drop following having intercourse. It just keeps going for a brief period, consequently, sex isn't consistently the treatment, since hypertension can be perilous to both you and your child, it's critical to work with your PCP to foster an arrangement to forestall or control it.

2 Labor and recovery are less troublesome

The compressions in your pelvic floor increment when you have a climax which assists with building the muscles you'll require for work and recuperation.

Whenever you've pushed your child through those muscles, they'll make some simpler memories developing" said Jeanne Faulkner, an enrolled medical caretaker, and creator of sound judgment pregnancy! Exploring a Head Pregnancy and Birth for Mother and Baby" in Portland, Oregon.

3 Stress alleviation

Even though pregnancy is normally a euphoric time, it's normal to be worried about your work, accounts, and how your life will change once your child has arrived. Oxytocin, the affection chemical delivered when you have a climax, can help you unwind and rest better.

4 Stronger ties

Having successive sex today will help to develop your close connection and bond with your life partner in the future just as construct a solid propensity. Interface with your accomplice while you have time since you require that association once the child is conceived.

5 Fewer visits to the bathroom

At any point do you want to go to the washroom? At the point when you're pregnant, you might have incessant excursions to the restroom just as spilling when you wheeze or snicker.

Baby grows bigger and rubs against your bladder. Similar muscles, you'll reinforce for work may likewise assist with pee stream.

6 preventing complication

Regular sex might assist with forestalling toxemia, as indicated by a Danish report. It's believed to be because of a protein contained in sperm that can handle the invulnerable arrangement of the body.

Notwithstanding, because the reason for toxemia is dubious, it's basic to keep the entirety of your pre-birth arrangement and examine your danger with your PCP.

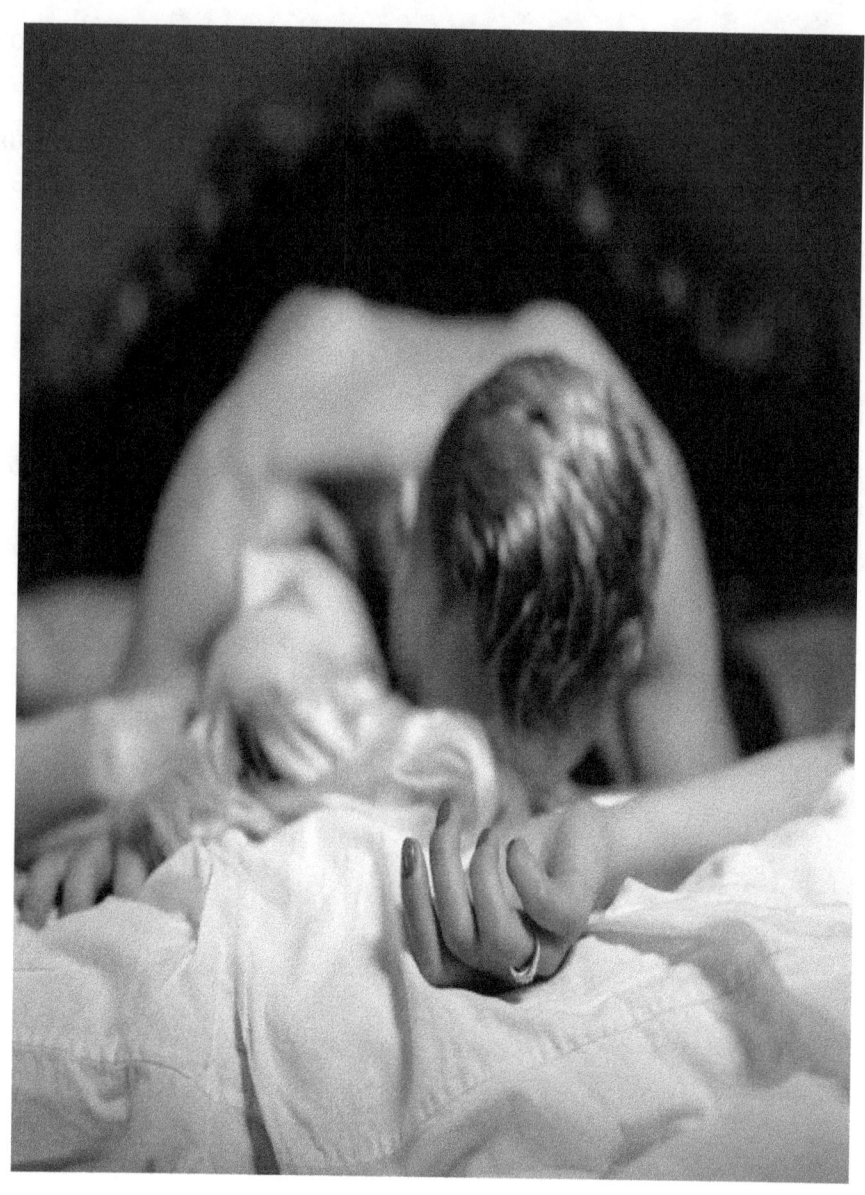

Chapter six

Fear of sex - what it causes, and outcomes

Assuming you leave in fear of intimacy, you likely think you are the only individual on the planet who experiences this issue yet you are not. indeed, it is assessed that around 4.5% of the people who visit sexology centers experience the ill effects of sex fear.

Assuming you continually stay away from sex, if sexual contact courses you stress or on the other hand when you find yourself being when your spouse kisses you or even comes close to you, all things considered, you have an abhorrence for closeness.

recognizing your concern is the first step

What is sex phobia?

people who feel repugnance for sex keep away from private contact with their partners and after some time might lose their sexual longing. Indeed, they may encounter an aversion towards intercourse as well as towards closeness, so that in the most outrageous cases they might dismiss any sort of approach from their accomplice particularly assuming they accept it might have sexual implications, like kissing and touching.

Anxiety toward sex includes various sentiments, from dread to aversion, disdain, or tension concerning conduct that has sexual hints. At times, the general thought of cozy contact triggers these responses.

There are various kinds of dismissal

1. You have consistently been having weird feelings about intimacy

2. You just experience the fear of intimacy with a specific companion

3. Post-traumatic. The individual has emerged because of a traumatic encounter connected to sexuality

This sort of sexual fear is more normal in ladies. Indeed, now and again, the aversion center focuses on explicit parts of sex, like a vaginal entrance or genital emissions. Certain individuals experience just mid nervousness, yet others experience extraordinary mental pain. In the further developed stages, fits of anxiety, swooning, queasiness, unsteadiness, and breathing challenges might happen. Unreasonable, yet you actually can't handle the staggering longing to avoid circumstances that might include cozy contact.

As a result, you are likely to use different strategies to avoid this situation, for example, going to bed too early or too late, dismissing your appearance to be ugly, or keeping yourself excessively occupied.

Reasons inspired by a paranoid fear of sex

The reasons inspired by a paranoid fear of intimacy are different, among the most well-known are the rigid and puritanical upbringing.

Inflexible and rigid childhood. By and large, behind the fear of sex lies a family background of sexual constraint. These are individuals who were educated as children that closeness was something negative or "grimy", so they have fostered a profound abhorrence for closeness in a couple's relationship.

Horrible sexual encounters. Now and again, the apprehension about closeness is the consequence of an unsavory encounter, either in sex or because the individual has been a casualty of assault or misuse.

Sexual brokenness. Now and then, sex fear is established in a sexual issue that makes closeness undesirable or even difficult like vaginismus or dyspareunia (agonizing intercourse} now and again, anorgasmia, untimely discharge, or erectile brokenness can likewise prompt a reduction in want or even an abhorrence for closeness.

Notwithstanding the abovementioned, there are a few factors that fuel dread of closeness, for example, relationship issues, feeling awkward with one's body, having low confidence, experiencing tension or despondency, or love OCD, creating ridiculous assumptions regarding sex, or bringing terrified of getting pregnant.

It has additionally been tracked down that individuals with the feeling of fear toward closeness, are bound to encounter various circumstances as undermining, although they are not, what happens is that you concentrate on the inconvenience, rather than zeroing in on partaking in the relationship continually watching your response, you add additional pressure that impedes delight.

In this present situation, the thoughtful sensory system is enforced because it has seen a danger. Subsequently, your breathing rate builds, you begin perspiring, your muscles worry and you feel your heart thumping quicker. It is difficult to have pleasurable intercourse in this state, so you steadily distinguish closeness from something negative.

Results of sex dismissal

Everybody is unique and suddenly encounters this issue. Nonetheless, assuming you fear sex, you are probably going to feel inadequate and live in an extremely durable condition of nervousness because, from one perspective, you might need to have an ordinary sexual coexistence, at the same time, then again, you additionally feel apprehensive.

Indeed, it is an exceptionally restricting sexual problem, as it doesn't just influence the sexual level. We can't fail to remember that what recognizes a couple's relationship is definitively that snapshot of closeness that permits the two individuals to get along and hold each other together. That is the reason, when sexual relations, become an issue, clashes regularly emerge in the couple too.

At the point when the problem is extreme, the individual dodges circumstances that include connecting with possible accomplices. In different cases, they get into an endless loop of separations, because as the level of intimacy assuming the relationship builds, they can't stand it and bring it up. This keeps them from keeping up with dependable heartfelt connections.

Chapter seven

Genophobia (fear of sex or sexual intimacy)

Side effects

Causes

Treatment

See a specialist

The feeling of fear towards sex or sexual intimacy is likewise called "xenophobia" or "erotophobia." This is more than a straightforward abhorrence or repugnance. A condition can cause extraordinary dread or frenzy when sexual intimacy endeavors. For certain, individuals, in any event, contemplating it can cause these sentiments.

There are different fears connected with Genophobia that may happen simultaneously:

nosophobia: the feeling of fear toward getting an illness or infection

gymnophobia: fear about nakedness (seeing others stripped, being seen bare, or both)

heterophobia: fear about the other gender

coitophobia: fear about intercourse

haphephobia: fear about being contacted just as contacting others

tocophobia: fear about pregnancy or labor

An individual may likewise have general dread or nervousness about being sincerely close with someone else. This can then convert into fear of sexual intimacy.

Indications of **Genophobia**

Fears include a more checked response than disliking or fearing something. By definition, fears include serious dread or uneasiness. They cause physical and mental responses that ordinarily disrupt ordinary working.

This dread response is set off by the occasion or circumstance that some individuals fear.

Ordinary phobic responses include:

a quick sensation of fear, nervousness, and frenzy when presented to the wellspring of the fear or even musings of the source (for this situation, a sexual experience)

an agreement that the dread is abnormal and outrageous in any case, simultaneously, a failure to limit it

a deteriorating of manifestations if the trigger isn't taken out

evasion of the circumstance that causes the dread response

sickness, tipsiness, inconvenience breathing, heart palpitations, or perspiring when presented to the trigger

Reasons for **Genophobia**

It isn't in every case clear what causes fears, even explicit fears. Assuming there is a particular reason, treating that cause initially is significant. Different reasons for **Genophobia** may incorporate physical or intense subject matters:

Vaginismus is the point at which the muscles of the vagina grip up automatically when vaginal infiltration endeavors. This can make intercourse agonizing or even unimaginable. It can likewise disrupt embedding a tampon. Such serious and reliable agony can prompt anxiety toward sexual closeness.

Erectile brokenness. Erectile brokenness (ED) is having difficulty or trouble acquiring and controlling an erection. Even though it's treatable, it may prompt sensations of humiliation, disgrace, or stress. Somebody with ED might not have any desire to impart this to someone else. Contingent upon how exceptional the sentiments are; this may make an individual unfortunate of sexual closeness.

Past sexual maltreatment or PTSD. children misuse or sexual maltreatment can cause post-awful pressure issues (PTSD) and influence how you view closeness or sex. It can likewise influence sexual work. While only one out of every odd overcomer of misuse creates PTSD or an apprehension about sex or closeness, these things may be a piece of certain people's feeling of dread toward sex.

Anxiety toward sexual execution. Certain individuals are anxious with regards to whether they're "great" in bed. This can cause extraordinary mental inconvenience, driving them to keep away from sexual closeness by and large because of a paranoid fear of scorn or lackluster showing.

Body disgrace or **dysmorphia.** The disgrace of one's body, just as being excessively hesitant with regards to the body, can adversely affect sexual fulfillment and cause tension. A few people with serious body disgrace or **dysmorphia** (considering the body to be imperfect even though, to others, it looks ordinary) may stay away from or dread sexual closeness through and through in light of the absence of joy and exceptional disgrace it brings them.

A past filled with assault. Assault or rape can cause PTSD and different sorts of sexual brokenness, incorporating negative relationships with sex. This may make somebody foster apprehension about sexual closeness.

Treatment for **Genophobia**

Assuming there is an actual part present, for example, **Vaginismus**, this can be dealt with appropriately. Torment with intercourse is normal. Whenever left untreated, it may prompt a dread or aversion to sex.

Assuming that an actual reason is recognized, treatment relies upon the particular issue, and afterward, any going with enthusiastic part can be tended to.

Treatment for fears commonly incorporates psychotherapy. Different sorts of psychotherapy have been demonstrated to be advantageous for fears, including mental conduct treatment (CBT) and openness treatment.

CBT includes dealing with creating elective perspectives about the fear or circumstance while likewise learning strategies to address actual responses to the trigger. It tends to be matched with openness to the dreaded circumstance (in a "schoolwork task," for instance).

A sex specialist can likewise be useful for tending to Genophobia. The sort of treatment in individual meetings relies generally upon the basic reasons for the fear and the particular circumstance.

When to see a specialist

The contrast between a gentle dread and a fear is that a fear contrarily affects your life, influencing it in huge ways. Feeling of dread toward sex can disrupt creating heartfelt connections. It can likewise add to sensations of seclusion and sorrow. Fears are treatable with treatment or potentially drug, contingent upon the circumstance.

A specialist can do a test to check whether there is an actual part to your apprehension about sex, and assuming this is the case, assist with treating that. Assuming that there is no basic actual angle, your primary care physician can give you assets and references to advisors who have practical experience in fears.

This condition is treatable. It isn't something you need to confront alone.

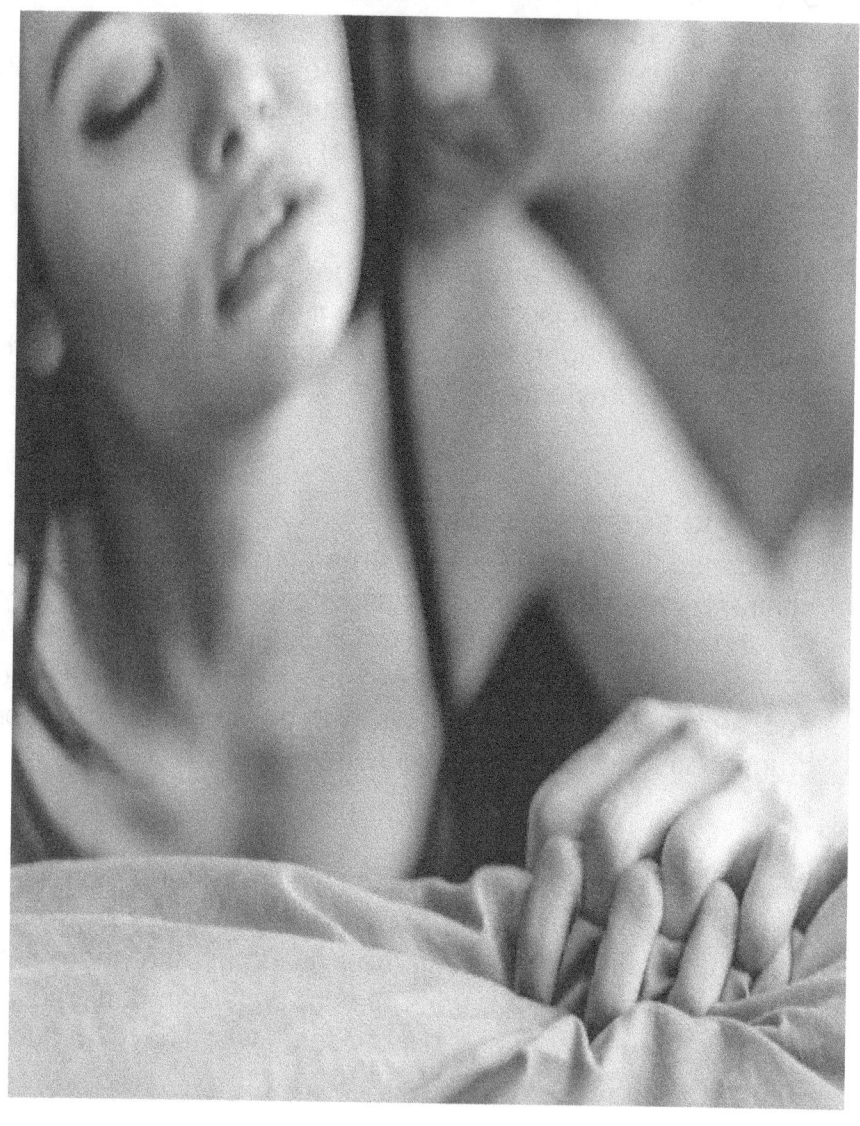

Chapter eight

Diagnosing fear of intimacy

It's generally really smart, to begin with, a total actual exam, particularly on the off chance that you haven't had one in some time. When actual sicknesses have been precluded, a specialist can allude you to fitting emotional wellness trained professional.

Specialists and therapists are prepared to direct assessments and analyze nervousness issues like the feeling of fear toward intimacy or avoidant behavioral condition.

Beating trepidation of intimacy

Your way to deal with beating these feelings of trepidation relies upon why you have them in any case, just as how serious the fear is.

You might have an extremely gentle fear that you can manage all alone or with some social treatment. Be that as it may, assuming your fear is because of injury, is extreme, or is joined by melancholy, proficient directing is suggested.

Grappling with your apprehension about intimacy

Ponder occasions in your day-to-day existence and attempt to get where your feelings of trepidation come from. Might it be said that you are unknowingly annihilating connections? Furthermore, do you need more significant connections?

Esteem yourself
All connections accompany a level of vulnerability. Many personal connections merit having, regardless of whether they keep going forever.

Give yourself a little room to breathe: You're flawed, yet not is any potential relationship accomplice. If somebody cuts off a friendship with you, it says nothing regarding your worth personally.

Impart
Open up to your partner. On the off chance that it's not excessively difficult, talk about your fear and where they come from. Assuming it's too difficult to even think about examining, disclose that you're willing to manage these issues with a clinical expert.

Characterize your limits. Depict what assists you with having a good sense of reassurance, just as things that trigger fear. Let your partner know what you want and let them in on your attempt to defeat your feelings of fear.

Look for help from an expert
The primary treatment for avoidant behavioral conditions is psychotherapy. Emotional psychotherapist can assist you to rectify where those apprehensions begin and how to control them.

At the point when your partner fears intimacy

Assuming it's your partner who has apprehension about intimacy, keep the lines of communication open. Tell them you're free to tune in, however, don't drive them into uncovering the wellspring of their feelings of trepidation. This might be excessively excruciating.

Support them in looking for treatment. Ask how you might assist them with having a good sense of reassurance. Show restraint, since figuring out how to adapt takes time. It's difficult, however, to remember that their feeling of fear toward intimacy isn't about you.

Focus point

If you feel frightened when it comes to intimacy, it means you have an emotional wellness problem that can lead you to disrupt connections and disconnect yourself. It requires some investment and persistence, yet with proficient direction, you can figure out how to beat your feelings of fear and structure significant bonds with others.

Execution Anxiety Doesn't Mean the End of Your Sex Life... Here's Why

Once in while sex can be distressing, yet these means might assist you with getting your section back.

After her first sexual accomplice put down her in the room, Steph Valarie started re-thinking herself when it came to sex.

"I felt afraid and uncertain about being a mistake to the next person," the 37-year-old says. "I ended up hating the feeling of intimacy and never wanting to have anything to do with engaging in sexual relations."

Indeed, even with various accomplices, Valarie "made a halfhearted effort" of sex, continuously trusting the demonstration would be over rapidly.

"I felt broken," she concedes. "What's more than whatever else, I felt even more awful about the negative feelings I felt with regards to sex. I felt that I wasn't somebody who merited focusing on. Then, at that point, I would feel angry for the way that I needed to feel remorseful and would need sex even less. It was an endless loop."

"Sex nervousness," like Valarie experienced, is anything but an authority clinical finding. It's a casual term used to portray dread or fear connected with sex. Yet, it is genuine - and it influences a larger number of individuals than is usually known.

"It has also been recorded, [the percentage] is generally high," says Michael J. Salas, LPC-S, AASECT, and affirmed sex specialist and relationship master in Dallas, Texas. It was also estimated that "Numerous sexual dysfunctions are generally normal, and practically all of the sexual brokenness cases that I've worked with have a component of nervousness related with them."

How sex uneasiness shows can happen in a wide assortment of ways for various individuals. Ladies might have a critical drop in moxie or interest, experience difficulty getting stirred or having a climax, or experience actual agony during sex. Men can battle with their exhibition or their capacity to discharge.

Certain individuals get so apprehensive at engaging in sexual relations that they try not to have it by and large.

Notwithstanding, Ravi Shah, MD, a specialist at Columbia Doctors and aide educator of psychiatry at Columbia University Medical Center in New York City, proposes one of the keys to defeating sex tension is seeing it as a "side effect" rather than a condition.

"when You're always getting nervous whenever it comes to sex, yet what's the genuine analysis?" Shah inquires.

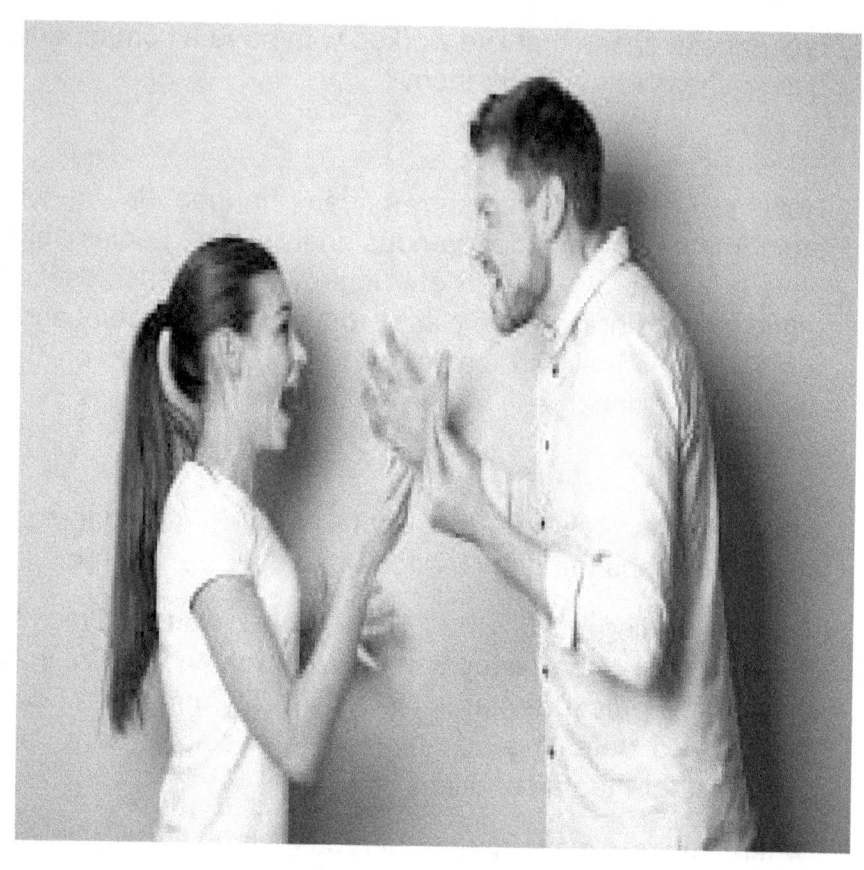

Chapter nine
The connection between uneasiness and sex

Assuming it seems like pretty much everybody you know is restless with regards to something nowadays - all things considered, that is because they are. Tension issues are as of now the most widely recognized psychological wellness issue in the United States, influencing around 40 million grown-ups.

At the point when an individual detects a danger (genuine or envisioned), their body intuitively switches into "acute stress" mode. Would it be advisable for me to remain and battle the snake before me, or book it to wellbeing?

The synthetics that get delivered into the body during this cycle don't add to Trusted Source sexual craving. For, they set a damper on it, so an individual's consideration can be centered around the quick danger.

"By and large, individuals who experience tension problems in the other lives are bound to encounter sexual brokenness, as well," says Nicole Prause, Ph.D., a sexual psych physiologist and authorized analyst in Los Angeles.

Also, injury - like sexual maltreatment or rape - can trigger anxiety about sex. So can constant torment, an adjustment of chemicals (like just after conceiving an offspring or while going through menopause), and surprisingly an absence of value sex schooling.

"Abstinence-only education, in general, try to create a stigma and disgrace around sex that can proceed into youthfulness and adulthood," says Salas. "Sex education centers focus more on pregnancy overlooks the significance of sexual excitement and joy. This can leave individuals seeking pornography for their sex training... [which] can build legends of sexual execution and increment tension."

"Certain individuals might have tension around sex since they have ridiculous assumptions regarding what sound sex is," concurs Shah. "Across all kinds of people, that has to do with low confidence, what sex resembles in pornography and motion pictures versus, in actuality, and how much sex they believe they 'ought to be having."

"there are people that goes with the idea that every other person is having intercourse all the time and it's incredible that they don't encounter issues aside from them," he adds.

how to lighten sex tension?

There are a lot of advantages to keeping a solid sexual coexistence. Sex works on your bond with your accomplice gives your confidence a lift and can bring down your circulatory strain and reinforce your invulnerable framework.

The "vibe great" chemicals delivered during sex can even assist with combatting sensations of stress and uneasiness.

So how would you move beyond your present nervousness about sex to receive those rewards?

Converse with your primary care physician
To begin with, preclude any actual issues.

"people who have violent behavior can build up sexual abuse, which can then expand sexual anxiety," Salas says. These incorporate constant medical problems like joint inflammation, malignant growth, and diabetes. Certain drugs, like antidepressants, can likewise decimate your drive.

Investigate intimacy in various ways
"Sensate Focus" works out, which include contacting your accomplice and being contacted for your pleasure, are intended to help you reconnect with both your sexy and sexual sentiments.

"in the first place, no genital contacting is permitted," explains Prause. "More heartbreaks is continuously added back in as life advance, which is frequently finished with a specialist between home meetings. These are done to assist with recognizing sources and seasons of nervousness and work through what those may mean."

Since tension "most frequently is tied in with something coming up short around the snapshots of the entrance," says Prause, you could likewise decide to stay away from that particular demonstration until your certainty works back. That way, you can figure out how to appreciate other pleasurable sexual exercises that give closeness, however without the tension.

Simply ensure you talk with your accomplice on the off chance that you conclude this course is best for you. As Prause alerts, "There's no avoiding great communication on this one."

Be careful

During sex, you might end up attempting to guess what your accomplice might be thinking or stressing that you're not satisfying their dreams. "Care can assist with keeping you in the present while overseeing gloomy feelings as they emerge," says Salas.

To do that, he asks his customers to see the signs they get from their bodies as data, rather than decisions. "Pay attention to your body, instead of attempting to supersede it," he says.

For example, rather than stressing why you don't yet have an erection - and freezing that you ought to - acknowledge that you're getting a charge out of how you're at present treating, kissing, or being moved by your accomplice.

"Seeing without being judgmental rather having acknowledgment are key parts of bringing down sexual nervousness," says Salas.

Make sex a customary discussion
"It's a dream that your partner should know what you need," says Shah. " most times they don't have the slightest idea of what you might need for supper without you saying it to them, and the equivalent goes for sexual activity."

Pick a private second and propose, "There's something I need to converse with you about concerning sex. Can we be able to deliberate that now?" This delicate heads-up will give your accomplice a second to intellectually plan. Then, at that point, approach the main issue: "I love you and need us to have a decent sexual coexistence. One thing that is difficult for me is [fill-in-the-blank]."

Remember to welcome your accomplice to ring in, as well, by inquiring: "How would you think our sexual coexistence is?"

Speaking transparently about sex might feel abnormal from the beginning, yet can be an extraordinary beginning stage for dealing with your uneasiness, Shah says.

Try not to limit foreplay

"There are various ways of getting sexual pleasure," says Shah. "massages, showers, manual masturbation, simply kissing and romancing each other... Build up a collection of good, positive encounters."

Investigate issues of disgrace

Perhaps you're humiliated with regards to your appearance, the number of accomplices you've had, a physically communicated infection - or maybe you were raised to accept that your sexuality is off-base.

"With regards to sex, disgrace isn't exceptionally a long way behind," says Salas. "The issue with disgrace is that we don't discuss it. A few of us will not possess it." Identify which viewpoint is making you feel embarrassed, then, at that point, think about opening up regarding it to your accomplice.

"At the point when individuals endure sharing the data that they're generally embarrassed about, the feelings of dread of sharing it diminish," says Salas. "They understand that they can share this, and still be acknowledged and adored."

Look for proficient assistance

On the off chance that your uneasiness isn't bound to the room, or you've attempted without progress to further develop your sexual coexistence, look for proficient assistance. "You might require more vigorous treatment with a specialist or even drug," says Shah.

HEALTHLINE CHALLENGE

What can you be able to achieve in a month without liquor?

It's never an awful ideal opportunity to monitor your relationship with liquor. Alcohol should be taken in moderately at least once in a month with the drawn-out Alcohol Reset Challenge.

Facing everyday life after sexual uneasiness

Steph Valarie didn't seek for solutions for her sex uneasiness. It stayed close by for a considerable length of time. In any event, when she met her present spouse, their first sexual experience was set apart by Valarie's tears and an admission that she had "abnormality" about sex.

A coincidental vocation as a sex writer assisted her with gradually beginning to understand that her uneasiness wasn't strange. "Individuals would remark or email me saying thanks to me for being so transparent with regards to a thing they were likewise encountering," says Valarie, who's currently composed a diary, "A Dirty Word," about her experience. "They had consistently had the view that they were facing their present predicament alone. Be that as it may, not even one of us are distant from everyone else in this."

At the point when she and her spouse choose to have a child, Valarie was astonished to observe that the more she engaged in sexual relations, the more she wanted it. A standard yoga practice additionally assisted her with working on a feeling of care, and she began asking her significant other for more foreplay and nonsexual closeness for the day.

"I likewise turned out to be more open to closeness in any event, when I wasn't really 'in the disposition.' Although we should be genuine," Valarie adds, "in some cases, I'm truly not in the state of mind, I honor that."

Also regarding our feelings is frequently the first (and greatest) venture toward beating sex uneasiness.

Conclusion

Sex is a significant piece of life and generally speaking, prosperity seeing someone, climaxes have a critical influence in holding. Physical and passionate advantages like decreased danger of coronary illness worked on confidence, and more can emerge out of engaging in sexual relations

You can in any case have comparable advantages without sex. Taking part in other pleasurable exercises like working out, collaborating with a pet, and having a solid organization of companions might offer similar advantages.

Sex can be used as an avenue to work on your fulfillment.

In any case, assuming sex is essential for your life, because of a relationship or want, it's critical to have the option to impart and encounter sexual fulfillment, you might find alleviation and an increment in bliss when you invest in some opportunity to have intercourse.

55

www.ingramcontent.com/pod-product-compliance
Lightning Source LLC
Chambersburg PA
CBHW070135230526
45472CB00004B/1536